SELF CARE FOR TEENS WITH ADHD

ADHD Teen Toolkit Nurturing Your Mind and Body through Self Care

By

William Davis

TABLE OF CONTENT

- Incorporating screen-free activities into daily routine
- Practicing digital wellness for better mental health

Coping with Emotional Regulation

- Understanding the emotional challenges faced by teens with ADHD
- Developing healthy coping mechanisms for emotional regulation
- Identifying triggers and managing emotions effectively
- Seeking support when needed

Seeking Professional Help

- Knowing when to seek professional help
- Understanding the different types of therapy for ADHD
- Working with counselors or therapists for support

- Incorporating professional help as part
  of self-care routine

CONCLUSION

Introduction

Consideration Shortfall/Hyperactivity Problem (ADHD) is a neurodevelopmental problem that influences a great many teenagers around the world. It is described by persevering examples of obliviousness, hyperactivity, and impulsivity that can essentially influence a youngster's day to day existence, including their scholarly presentation, social connections, and close to home prosperity. ADHD is a mind boggling condition with different subtypes, including dominatingly unmindful sort, overwhelmingly hyperactive-indiscreet sort, and consolidated type.

In pre-adulthood, the side effects of ADHD might be introduced in one of a kind ways, and it very well may be trying for both the teenagers and their families to explore the intricacies of this condition during this basic formative stage. It is essential to acquire a more profound comprehension of ADHD in youngsters to successfully uphold their necessities and advance their general prosperity.

CHAPTER 1

What is ADHD in Teens?

ADHD is a neurobiological condition that influences the chief elements of the mind, including the capacity to direct consideration, impulsivity, and restraint. In teenagers, these side effects might show diverse contrasts with more youthful youngsters, as the requests of puberty increment with scholastic obligations, social connections, and hormonal changes.

Common Symptoms of ADHD in Teens

Youngsters with ADHD might show a scope of side effects that can influence different parts of their life, including:

1. Absentmindedness: Teenagers with ADHD might battle with focusing on subtleties, supporting consideration in undertakings or exercises, arranging errands, and adhering to guidelines or finishing tasks.

2. Hyperactivity: While hyperactivity might diminish in puberty contrasted with youth, teenagers with ADHD might in any case encounter fretfulness, squirming, and trouble participating in peaceful or quiet exercises.

3. Impulsivity: Adolescents with ADHD might experience issues controlling motivations, bringing about hasty direction, interfering with others, and participating in dangerous ways of behaving.

4. Scholastic Difficulties: ADHD can influence a high schooler's scholarly presentation, incorporating troubles with arranging, focusing on, and finishing tasks, as well as difficulties with using time productively and considering.

5. Profound Dysregulation: Youngsters with ADHD might battle with close to home guidelines, encountering emotional episodes, crabbiness, disappointment, and hardships overseeing pressure and tension.

Challenges Faced by Teens with ADHD
Youngsters with ADHD might confront different difficulties that can influence their day to day existence, including:

1. Scholarly and Instructive Difficulties: ADHD side effects can adversely influence a high schooler's scholastic presentation, prompting lower grades, inadequate tasks, and troubles with using time productively and association.

2. Social and Relational Difficulties: Youngsters with ADHD might battle with shaping and keeping up with sound connections, as they might experience issues with motivation control, profound guideline, and interactive abilities.

3. Profound and Emotional wellness Difficulties: ADHD can essentially influence a high schooler's close to home prosperity, prompting expanded hazard of creating state of mind problems, uneasiness, and low confidence.

4. Unsafe Ways of behaving: Impulsivity and unfortunate motivation control related with ADHD might prompt taking part in dangerous ways of behaving, for example, substance misuse, foolish driving, and other rash activities with possible long haul results.

5. Co-happening Conditions: Adolescents with ADHD might have an expanded gamble of creating co-happening conditions, for example, learning disabilities, mind-set issues, nervousness problems, and oppositional rebellious turmoil (ODD), which can additionally entangle their psychological well-being and prosperity.

Importance of self-care for teens with ADHD

Taking care of oneself assumes a significant part in overseeing ADHD side effects and advancing by and large prosperity in youngsters. By understanding the novel difficulties looked by youngsters with ADHD and carrying out viable procedures, teenagers can figure out how to adapt to their side effects, work on their profound guidelines, upgrade their scholastic exhibition, and foster sound social connections.

CHAPTER 2

Managing Medication

Working with a healthcare professional

Working with a healthcare professional is an essential aspect of maintaining good health and managing any medical conditions. Whether you're seeking routine care, managing a chronic illness, or dealing with an acute health issue, establishing a productive and collaborative relationship with your healthcare provider is crucial. Here's a complete and detailed guide on how to work effectively with a healthcare professional.

1. Choose the Right Healthcare Professional: The first step in working with a healthcare professional is to choose the right one for your needs. Consider the type of healthcare provider you need, such as a primary care physician, specialist, or therapist, based on your specific health concerns. Look for healthcare professionals who are licensed, experienced, and reputable. Consider their qualifications, expertise,

and communication style to ensure a good fit for your healthcare needs.

2. Prepare for Appointments: Before your appointment, take some time to prepare. Make a list of your symptoms, concerns, and questions. Write down any medications, supplements, or treatments you are currently taking. Be prepared to provide your healthcare professional with your complete medical history, including past surgeries, allergies, and family medical history. Having this information readily available will help your healthcare provider make an accurate diagnosis and develop an appropriate treatment plan.

3. Establish Open Communication: Effective communication is essential in any healthcare relationship. Be open and honest with your healthcare professional about your symptoms, concerns, and lifestyle habits. Provide accurate information about your medical history and disclose any relevant information, even if it may be uncomfortable or embarrassing. Be an

active participant in your healthcare by asking questions, seeking clarification, and expressing any concerns you may have. Clear and open communication will help your healthcare provider understand your needs and provide appropriate care.

4. Follow Treatment Plans: Once your healthcare professional has developed a treatment plan, it's important to follow it diligently. This may include taking medications as prescribed, following dietary restrictions, engaging in regular physical activity, or attending appointments for tests or therapies. It's crucial to adhere to the treatment plan to achieve the best possible health outcomes. If you have any concerns or difficulties with your treatment plan, discuss them openly with your healthcare provider, and work together to find solutions.

5. Educate Yourself: Educating yourself about your health condition and treatment options is empowering. Take the initiative to learn about your diagnosis, treatment options, and

possible side effects. Ask your healthcare professional for reliable sources of information or educational materials. However, be cautious with information from the internet or other sources, and always verify the information with your healthcare provider to ensure accuracy.

6. Advocate for Yourself: You are your best advocate in your healthcare journey. If you have concerns or questions about your care, don't hesitate to speak up. Ask for clarification if you don't understand something, and express your preferences and concerns to your healthcare provider. Remember that you have the right to be actively involved in your healthcare decisions and to make informed choices about your treatment.

7. Follow-up and Monitor Your Health: After your initial appointment, it's important to follow-up with your healthcare provider as recommended. Regular check-ups and follow-up appointments allow your healthcare provider to monitor your progress, make adjustments to your treatment plan if necessary, and address any concerns or

questions you may have. Keep track of your symptoms, changes in your health, and any side effects from medications or treatments. If you notice any changes or have concerns, contact your healthcare provider promptly.

8. Be Respectful and Trust Your Healthcare Professional: Building a trusting and respectful relationship with your healthcare provider is essential. Remember that they are experts in their field and have your best interests at heart. Respect their expertise, recommendations, and decisions, and trust their judgment. If you have doubts or concerns, discuss them openly and respectfully with your healthcare provider. Trusting your healthcare professional and maintaining open communication will foster a collaborative relationship and lead to better healthcare outcomes.

9. Involve Caregivers or Family Members if Applicable: If you have a caregiver or family member who is involved in your healthcare, make sure to include them in your healthcare journey. They can

provide support, help you remember important information, and be an additional resource for communication with your healthcare provider. Make sure to provide your healthcare provider with appropriate consent to involve your caregivers or family members in your care, if applicable.

10. Take Responsibility for Your Own Health: While your healthcare professional plays a crucial role in managing your health, ultimately, you are responsible for your own health. Take ownership of your health by making healthy lifestyle choices, following your treatment plan, attending appointments, and actively participating in your healthcare decisions. Remember that healthcare is a partnership between you and your healthcare provider, and your active engagement in your own health is vital.

11. Be Patient and Realistic: Managing health conditions or achieving health goals may take time and effort. Be patient with yourself and with your healthcare provider. Understand that healthcare is a complex field, and not all

issues may be resolved quickly or with immediate results. Set realistic expectations and communicate openly with your healthcare provider about your progress, challenges, and concerns.

12. Seek Second Opinions if Needed: If you have doubts or concerns about your diagnosis or treatment plan, don't hesitate to seek a second opinion from another qualified healthcare professional. Getting a second opinion can provide you with additional perspectives and information to make informed decisions about your health. Discuss your intention to seek a second opinion with your primary healthcare provider, as they can provide recommendations and help coordinate the process.

13. Keep Your Healthcare Provider Informed: As your health status changes, make sure to keep your healthcare provider informed. If you experience new symptoms, changes in your medication regimen, or any other relevant health changes, update your healthcare provider during

appointments or through appropriate communication channels. Keeping your healthcare provider informed ensures that your treatment plan can be adjusted as needed to provide you with the best possible care.

14. Respect Privacy and Confidentiality: Healthcare providers are bound by strict confidentiality and privacy laws. Respect the privacy and confidentiality of your healthcare provider by not sharing your personal health information with others without proper consent. Similarly, ensure that you provide accurate and complete information to your healthcare provider, as this is essential for accurate diagnosis and treatment planning.

Understanding the medication regimen

1. Understanding your drug routine is a significant part of working with a medical care proficient. Meds are frequently recommended as a feature of a treatment intended to oversee medical issues or side effects. Here are a few central issues to remember with regards to figuring out your medicine routine:

2. Know the Names and Motivations behind Your Meds: Ensure you know the names of the multitude of drugs you are taking, including both remedy and non-prescription meds, as well as any nutrients or enhancements. Comprehend the motivation behind every prescription and the way things are supposed to help your wellbeing. Request that your medical care supplier make sense of any medicine that you are muddled about.

3. Figure out Measurements and Guidelines: Be know about the doses and directions for taking every medicine. Follow the recommended measurements and organization directions cautiously, including the recurrence, timing, and length of every drug. Assuming you have any different kinds of feedback about how to take your drugs, counsel your medical care supplier or drug specialist for explanation.

4. Know about Likely Aftereffects: Prescriptions can make side impacts,

which are critical to know about. Comprehend the likely symptoms of every prescription you are taking, and know what to look for. Assuming you experience any surprising or extreme incidental effects, advise your medical services supplier right away.

5. Know the Connection with Different Meds: A few drugs can cooperate with one another, prompting possible unfavorable impacts or decreased viability. Illuminate your medical services supplier pretty much every one of the meds, nutrients, and enhancements you are taking, including any progressions or increments, to guarantee that there are no potential medication communications.

6. Get some information about Elective Choices: In the event that you have worries about the prescriptions you are taking, like possible secondary effects or connections, or on the other hand assuming you like to investigate elective treatment choices, examine these worries with your medical care supplier. They can give you data about elective

prescriptions or treatment choices that might be reasonable for your ailment.

7. Keep a Prescription Rundown: Keep a refreshed rundown of the relative multitude of drugs you are taking, including the names, measurements, and organization directions. This rundown can be useful for reference during meetings with your medical care supplier, if there should be an occurrence of crises, or while seeing new medical services suppliers. Make a point to likewise illuminate your parental figures or relatives, if pertinent, about your prescription rundown.

8. Follow the Medicine Timetable: Stick to your drug plan as recommended by your medical care supplier. Skipping dosages or taking prescriptions conflictingly can influence their adequacy. Assuming that you experience issues making sure to take your prescriptions, consider setting updates or utilizing pill coordinators to assist you with keeping focused.

9. Convey Changes to Your Medical care Supplier: Illuminate your medical care

supplier about any progressions in your drug routine, including any new meds, changes in doses, or end of meds. This helps your medical care supplier to have a precise record of your drugs and make suitable acclimations to your therapy plan on a case by case basis.

10. Speak the truth About Medicine Use: Be straightforward with your medical care supplier about your prescription use, including any meds that are not endorsed, like non-prescription meds, natural enhancements, or sporting medications. This data is significant for your medical services supplier to have an extensive comprehension of your wellbeing and settle on informed conclusions about your consideration.

11. Seek clarification on some pressing issues: Go ahead and ask questions assuming that you have any worries or vulnerabilities about your medicine routine. Your medical services supplier is there to give you data and direction. Explain any questions or look for additional clarification about your meds

to guarantee that you completely
comprehend your treatment plan.

Remembering to take medication on time

Making sure to take drugs on time can be
testing, however it is vital for the adequacy of
your treatment plan. Here are a few hints to
assist you with remaining focused with taking
as much time as necessary:

1. Set Updates: Use alerts, clocks, or
   portable applications to set suggestions
   to take your drugs at explicit times
   during the day. You can likewise utilize a
   schedule or a medicine tracker to
   separate each portion as you take it.

2. Use Pill Coordinators: Pill coordinators,
   otherwise called pillboxes or medicine
   coordinators, can be useful in keeping
   your prescriptions coordinated and
   guaranteeing that you require some
   investment. You can track down
   different sorts of pill coordinators, like
   everyday or week after week

coordinators with compartments for various times.

3. Regularly practice It: Integrate bringing your drug into your everyday daily schedule. For instance, take your drug simultaneously every day, for example, during a dinner or before sleep time, to assist with laying out a propensity.

4. Use Innovation: A huge number of smartwatches have medicine update applications that can send you notices when now is the ideal time to take your drugs. You can likewise utilize savvy pillboxes that interface with your telephone by means of Bluetooth and send updates when now is the ideal time to take your prescriptions.

5. Include a Guardian or Relative: In the event that you have a parental figure or relative who assists you with your medicine routine, enroll their assistance in reminding you to take as much time as necessary.

6. Keep Drugs Noticeable: Keep your meds where you can see them effectively, for

example, on your end table, washroom counter, or kitchen counter. This can act as a visual wake up call to take as much time as is needed.

7. Prepare: Ensure you have sufficient drugs available to go on until your next top off. Reorder your medicines on time to abstain from running out of drugs and missing portions.

8. Speak with Your Medical services Supplier: On the off chance that you find it hard to make sure to require your prescriptions on investment, examine it with your medical care supplier. They might have the option to recommend elective dosing timetables or techniques to assist you with recalling.

9. Try not to Skip Dosages: Attempt to accept your meds as recommended by your medical care supplier and try not to skip portions, regardless of whether you feel much improved or figure you don't require them. Skipping portions can influence the viability of your treatment.

10. Be Straightforward with Yourself: Be straightforward with yourself about your adherence to your drug plan. Assuming you find it trying to make sure to require your drugs on investment, recognize it and do whatever it may take to further develop your prescription daily schedule.

Managing potential side effects

Overseeing potential incidental effects is a significant part of any clinical treatment. On the off chance that you are encountering secondary effects from a medicine or clinical mediation, here are a few basic principles for overseeing them:

1. Adhere to Directions: Consistently adhere to the guidelines given by your medical care supplier or drug specialist for taking prescriptions or going through clinical therapies. This incorporates doses, recurrence, and any exceptional guidelines connected with food or drink.

2. Speak with Your Medical care Supplier:
    On the off chance that you experience
    any secondary effects, it's critical to
    speak with your medical care supplier at
    the earliest opportunity. They can give
    direction on the best way to deal with
    the aftereffects and may have to change
    your treatment plan if vital.

3. Screen Side effects: Monitor any
    aftereffects you experience, including
    their seriousness, length, and
    recurrence. This data can be useful while
    talking about your side effects with your
    medical care supplier.

4. Hydrate: Drinking a lot of water can
    assist with flushing out certain
    prescriptions from your framework and
    may ease specific secondary effects like
    dry mouth or blockage. It's essential to
    adhere to a particular rule given by your
    medical services supplier in regards to
    liquid admission.

5. Rest: A few incidental effects might
    cause weakness or tiredness. It's vital to
    get satisfactory rest and stay away from
    exercises that require sharpness, like

driving or working large equipment, assuming you are encountering such secondary effects.

6. Change Diet: at times, adjusting your eating routine might assist with overseeing secondary effects. For instance, in the event that you experience gastrointestinal side effects, for example, sickness or loose bowels, staying away from zesty or greasy food varieties might be valuable. It's ideal to talk with your medical services supplier or an enrolled dietitian for explicit dietary proposals.

7. Stay away from Liquor and Tobacco: Liquor and tobacco can associate with meds and fuel specific aftereffects. It's essential to keep away from or limit their utilization as exhorted by your medical services supplier.

8. Utilize Strong Measures: Contingent upon the secondary effect, you might track down help from utilizing steady measures, for example, applying a virus pack, utilizing over-the-counter painkillers (whenever permitted by your

medical care supplier), or involving skin creams or balms as coordinated.

9. Follow Security Insurances: On the off chance that you are going through a clinical treatment with possible incidental effects, it's critical to follow all wellbeing safeguards, like wearing defensive stuff, staying away from sun openness, or sticking to dietary or way of life limitations as exhorted by your medical care supplier.

10. Look for Crisis Clinical Consideration if necessary: In the event that you experience extreme or dangerous secondary effects, for example, trouble breathing, serious hypersensitive responses, or chest torment, look for guaranteed clinical consideration or call crisis administrations

CHAPTER 3

Creating Healthy Routines

Establishing regular sleep patterns

Laying out customary rest designs, otherwise called rehearsing great rest cleanliness, is significant for generally wellbeing and prosperity. Here are a few ways to lay out customary rest designs:

1. Adhere to a Reliable Rest Timetable: Attempt to head to sleep and awaken simultaneously consistently, even at the end of the week. This controls your body's inner clock, which can work on the nature of your rest.

2. Make a Loosening up Sleep time Schedule: Lay out a loosening up sleep time routine to indicate to your body that now is the ideal time to slow down. This might incorporate exercises like perusing a book, paying attention to quieting music, washing up, or rehearsing unwinding procedures like profound breathing or reflection.

3. Establish a Climate: Ensure your rest climate is helpful for great rest that welcomes rests. Keep your room cool, dull, and calm. Consider utilizing power outage shades, earplugs, or a repetitive sound to shut out any troublesome commotions.

4. Limit Openness to Gadgets Before Bed: The blue light discharged by screens on electronic gadgets can disrupt your body's creation of melatonin, a chemical that manages rest. Attempt to restrict your openness to hardware, for example, cell phones, tablets, and PCs, for essentially an hour prior to sleep time.

5. Stay away from Energizers Before Bed: Try not to consume energizers, for example, caffeine and nicotine near sleep time, as they can disrupt your capacity to nod off. Keeping away from caffeine and nicotine for something like 4-6 hours before bedtime is ideal.

6. Get Customary Activity: Ordinary actual work during the day can assist you with resting better around evening time. Simply be careful not to practice

excessively near sleep time, as it might invigorate your body and make it harder to nod off.

7. Limit Rests: While snoozing can be valuable, particularly for more seasoned grown-ups or the people who are sleepless, it's ideal to restrict rests to 20-30 minutes during the day and try not to rest excessively near sleep time, as it can obstruct your capacity to nod off around evening time.

8. Establish an Agreeable Rest Climate: Put resources into an agreeable bedding, cushions, and bedding to establish an agreeable rest climate that advances great rest. Try different things with various kinds of pads and sleeping cushion solidness levels to find what turns out best for you.

9. Oversee Pressure: Elevated degrees of stress can upset your rest designs. Practice pressure the executives procedures like care, unwinding methods, or conversing with a specialist assuming you're battling with pressure or tension that is influencing your rest.

10. Counsel a Medical services Supplier: On
the off chance that you're having
industrious rest troubles, counseling a
medical services supplier for assessment
and guidance is significant. They can
assist with recognizing any basic clinical
or rest problems and give suitable
treatment choices.

Planning and managing daily activities

Arranging and overseeing day to day exercises
can assist you with remaining coordinated,
decrease pressure, and further develop
efficiency. Here are a few hints for really
arranging and dealing with your day to day
exercises:

1. Make a Plan for the day: Begin every day
by making a daily agenda. Record every
one of the assignments you really want
to achieve for the afternoon, focusing on
them in view of significance and
earnestness. This can assist you with
remaining on track and coordinated
over the course of the day.

2. Put forth Savvy Objectives: Set Explicit, Quantifiable, Feasible, Significant, and Time-bound (Brilliant) objectives for your day to day exercises. This assists you with explaining what should be finished and gives an internal compass and inspiration.

3. Utilize a Schedule or Organizer: Use a schedule or organizer to plan your day to day exercises. Dole out unambiguous times for each undertaking or movement to guarantee you have an unmistakable arrangement and can deal with your time successfully.

4. Focus on Undertakings: Focus on your errands in view of their significance and earnestness. Center around finishing high-need undertakings first and abstain from getting overpowered by attempting to do everything simultaneously.

5. Break Undertakings into More modest Advances: Assuming you have bigger errands or tasks, break them into more modest, more reasonable advances. This can make them less overwhelming and

more straightforward to handle, assisting you with gaining ground and remaining roused.

6. Limit Interruptions: Limit interruptions while chipping away at your day to day exercises. Switch off notices on your telephone, close pointless tabs on your PC, and track down a tranquil, centered climate to work in, if conceivable.

7. Delegate or Re-appropriate Errands: Assuming you have the choice, delegate or rethink assignments that can be taken care of by others. This can assist with saving your significant investment for additional significant undertakings or exercises that require your consideration.

8. Be Adaptable and Adjust: Be ready to change your arrangements and adjust to startling changes or difficulties that might emerge during the day. Remain adaptable and modify your timetable on a case by case basis.

9. Enjoy Reprieves: Enjoying short reprieves over the course of the day can

help you re-energize and keep up with efficiency. Use breaks to rest, stretch, or take part in exercises that help you unwind and revive.

10. Practice Time Usage Strategies: Use time usage procedures like the Pomodoro Method (working in centered spans followed by brief breaks), time impeding (allotting explicit time allotments for assignments), or the Eisenhower Framework (classifying undertakings in view of desperation and significance) to really deal with your time.

Creating a study schedule

Making a review timetable can assist you with remaining coordinated, deal with your time really, and boost your learning and maintenance of data. Here are a few ways to make a viable review plan:

1. Survey Your Objectives and Needs:
   Begin by explaining your review
   objectives and needs. What subjects or
   points do you have to study? What are
   your cutoff times or test dates?
   Understanding your objectives and
   needs will assist you with making an
   engaged report plan.

2. Realize Your Learning Style: Consider
   your favored learning style while making
   your review plan. Do you learn best
   through visual, hear-able, or sensation
   strategies? Tailor your review timetable
   to integrate exercises that line up with
   your learning style for ideal
   maintenance of data.

3. Decide Accessible Review Time: Assess
   your day to day and week by week
   timetable to decide the accessible review
   time. Think about your responsibilities,
   like classes, work, extracurricular
   exercises, and individual obligations. Be
   sensible about the time you can devote
   to contemplating.

4. Separate Your Review Material:
   Separate your review material into more

modest, reasonable lumps. Make a rundown of points or sections that you really want to cover, and gauge the time expected for each. This will assist you with making a review plan that is feasible and not overpowering.

5. Make a Review Schedule: Lay out a review routine by dispensing explicit times for concentrating on your timetable. Consistency is critical, so expect to learn simultaneously every day or week to foster a propensity.

6. Be Adaptable and Practical: Be sensible about your review plan and consider adaptability. Life can be unusual, and unforeseen occasions or changes might expect acclimations to your review plan. Be ready to adjust and make changes depending on the situation.

7. Utilize Useful Review Strategies: Integrate successful review procedures into your timetable. This might incorporate dynamic perusing, note-taking, summing up data in a way that would sound natural to you, making cheat sheets, rehearsing self-testing, or

dealing with training issues. Explore different avenues regarding various methods and find what turns out best for you.

8. Enjoy Reprieves: Try not to pack for extended periods without breaks, as it can prompt burnout and decreased efficiency. Plan ordinary brief breaks during your review meetings to rest and re-energize.

9. Stay away from Performing multiple tasks: Stay away from performing multiple tasks during your review time, as it can diminish efficiency and maintenance of data. Center around each undertaking or subject in turn to take advantage of your review meetings.

10. Audit and Reexamine: Consistently survey and amend your review plan as you progress. Evaluate what is working and what needs improvement, and make vital changes in accordance with keeping focused.

Incorporating physical exercise into daily routine

Integrating actual activity into your day to day schedule is significant for keeping up with by and large wellbeing and prosperity. Ordinary actual work can assist with working on actual wellness, oversee pressure, support temperament, increment energy levels, and diminish the gamble of different medical issues. Here are a few ways to integrate actual activity into your everyday daily schedule:

1. Put forth Exercise Objectives: Begin by defining explicit activity objectives that are reasonable and reachable. This could be a sure number of steps each day, a particular length of activity, or a specific kind of actual work. Defining objectives can assist you with remaining roused and centered.

2. Pick Exercises You Appreciate: Find proactive tasks that you appreciate and are probably going to stay with. This could be strolling, running, cycling, swimming, moving, playing a game, or taking a wellness class. At the point

when you partake in the action, you are
bound to practice it regularly.

3. Plan Exercise Time: Deal with practice
    like some other arrangement on your
    schedule and timetable it into your day
    to day everyday practice. Pick a period of
    day that turns out best for yourself and
    make it a non-debatable piece of your
    daily schedule. It may very well be in the
    first part of the day, during your mid-
    day break, or at night, contingent upon
    your timetable and inclinations.

4. Be Imaginative with Your Current
    circumstance: Search for chances to be
    truly dynamic in your day to day daily
    schedule. For instance, use the stairwell
    rather than the lift, walk or bicycle to
    work or school, park farther away from
    your objective to get a few additional
    means, or do family errands that require
    actual exertion.

5. Split It Up: On the off chance that you
    lack the capacity to deal with a long
    exercise, have a go at breaking your
    activity into more limited, more
    successive meetings over the course of

the day. For instance, you can do a fast 10-minute exercise in the first part of the day, go for a lively stroll during your mid-day break, and do some bodyweight practices at night.

6. Make it Social: Exercise with a companion, relative, or an exercise pal to make it more charming and consider each other responsible. You can likewise join bunch wellness classes or sports associations to make practice a social movement.

7. Be Adaptable: Be adaptable with your work-out daily practice and adjust it to your changing timetable and conditions. On the off chance that you miss an exercise or can't do your standard activity, view elective ways as genuinely dynamic, like going for a stroll, doing a fast home exercise, or taking part in open air exercises.

8. Stand by listening to Your Body: Focus on your body's signs and abstain from propelling yourself excessively hard or overlooking indications of weariness or inconvenience. It's essential to practice

at a level that is protected and agreeable for you.

9. Remain Hydrated: Make sure to drink a lot of water previously, during, and after your activity meetings to remain hydrated and perform at your best.

10. Keep tabs on Your Development: Monitor your work-out daily schedule and progress. This can assist you with remaining persuaded and praise your accomplishments. Utilize a wellness application, a diary, or a straightforward bookkeeping sheet to record your exercises, steps, or other proactive tasks.

CHAPTER 4

Managing Time and Prioritizing Tasks

Strategies for managing time effectively

Using time effectively is a significant expertise for really adjusting the requests of day to day existence, including work, school, individual errands, and relaxation exercises. Here are a few systems for overseeing time really:

1. Put forth Boundaries: Recognize the main undertakings and exercises that should be finished and focus on them. Utilize a plan for the day or an errand of the board instrument to monitor your undertakings and sort out them in view of their significance and cutoff time.

2. Prepare: Invest energy every day or week to prepare. Make a timetable or an everyday/week after week organizer that frames your errands and exercises for every day. This can assist you with remaining on track and coordinated, and forestall last-minute scrambling.

3. Break Errands into More modest
   Advances: Huge undertakings or
   activities can appear to be overpowering,
   so break them into more modest,
   reasonable advances. This can cause
   them to feel more feasible and assist you
   with gaining ground reliably.

4. Set Sensible Cutoff times: Be reasonable
   about how long undertakings require
   and set cutoff times in like manner. Try
   not to over-burden yourself with an
   excessive number of undertakings or
   setting unreasonable assumptions that
   can prompt pressure and frustration.

5. Take out or Delegate Trivial
   Undertakings: Recognize assignments
   that are not fundamental or can be
   designated to other people, and kill or
   represent them if conceivable. This can
   save additional opportunity for
   significant undertakings and exercises.

6. Keep away from Hesitation: Dawdling
   can prompt pointless pressure and
   deferrals. Attempt to defeat dawdling by
   breaking errands into more modest
   advances, setting cutoff times, utilizing

clocks or alerts, and utilizing procedures like the Pomodoro Strategy (working in centered overflows with brief breaks).

7. Limit Interruptions: Distinguish and limit interruptions that can gobble up your time, like web-based entertainment, messages, or superfluous interferences. Use efficiency instruments or methods like time obstructing to remain fixed on your undertakings.

8. Figure out how to Say No: It's essential to define limits and figure out how to express no to errands or exercises that don't line up with your needs or are impossible for you. Be aware of your limits and keep away from overcommitting yourself.

9. Practice Time Piecing: Time lumping includes gathering comparable undertakings or exercises and committing a particular time block for them. For instance, you can save a particular time block for browsing and answering messages, some other time

block for centered work, and one more
for exercise or taking care of oneself.

10. Enjoy Reprieves:Enjoying   ordinary
    reprieves can really assist   with further
    developing efficiency by lessening
    mental weakness and upgrading
    centers. Plan brief breaks during your
    day to rest,   re-energize, and stay
    balanced.

Prioritizing tasks and setting goals

Focusing on undertakings and defining
objectives are fundamental parts of viable
using time effectively. Here are a few
procedures for focusing on errands and laying
out objectives:

1. Distinguish Pressing versus Significant
   Undertakings: Pressing errands are
   those that require prompt consideration,
   while significant assignments are those
   that line up with your drawn out
   objectives and have huge effect. Focus
   on undertakings that are both dire and
   significant, as the need might arise to be
   tended to first.

2. Put forth Shrewd Objectives: Brilliant represents Explicit, Quantifiable, Attainable, Pertinent, and Time-bound. Set clear, explicit, and quantifiable objectives that are reachable inside a reasonable time period and line up with your needs.

3. Utilize a Need Framework: A need grid is a visual instrument that assists you with ordering undertakings in view of their desperation and significance. You can make a network with four quadrants: Earnest and Significant, Significant however not Dire, Critical yet not Significant, and Not Pressing or Significant. This can assist you with outwardly surveying and focus on undertakings in light of their significance and criticalness.

4. Think about Cutoff times: Consider cutoff times while focusing on assignments. Errands with approaching cutoff times might have to take need over different undertakings to guarantee opportune fruition.

5. Assess Advantages and Outcomes:
   Think about the possible advantages and
   results of finishing or not following
   through with a job. Errands that have
   high advantages or extreme results
   might be focused on in a like manner.

6. Survey and Once again focus on
   Consistently: Needs might change over
   the long haul, so it's critical to audit and
   once again focus on errands routinely.
   Be adaptable and change your needs
   founded on evolving conditions, new
   data, and moving objectives.

7. Stay away from Overcommitting: Be
   aware of taking on such a large number
   of undertakings immediately, as it can
   prompt overpower and diminished
   efficiency. Figure out how to say no
   when important and be practical about
   what you can reasonably achieve inside
   a given time span.

8. Center around High-Effect
   Undertakings: Recognize assignments
   that have the most elevated influence as
   far as accomplishing your objectives and
   spotlight on them. Focus on errands that

will draw you nearer to your ideal
results and line up with your drawn out
vision.

9. Break Errands into Reasonable
    Advances: Enormous undertakings or
    objectives can feel overpowering. Break
    them down into more modest, more
    reasonable advances that you can chip
    away at steadily. This can assist you with
    gaining ground and gather speed
    towards accomplishing your objectives.

10. Consider Your Energy Levels:
    Consider your energy levels and
    timetable errands likewise. Assuming
    you have high energy levels toward the
    beginning of the day, focus on
    significant and testing errands during
    that time, and leave less basic
    assignments for when your energy levels
    might plunge.

Using tools such as planners or apps for organization

Utilizing instruments like organizers or applications for association can enormously improve your capacity to really deal with your time. Here are a few systems for integrating organizers or applications into your hierarchical daily schedule:

1. Pick the Right Instrument: There are different kinds of organizers and applications accessible, so pick the one that best meets your requirements and inclinations. Consider factors, for example, the sort of errands you want to make due, your favored technique for association (e.g., advanced or paper-based), and the highlights presented by the instrument.

2. Set Up a Framework: Whenever you have picked an organizer or application, set up a framework for coordinating your errands and objectives inside it. This might include making classes or segments for various sorts of assignments (e.g., work, individual,

wellbeing, and so on), setting up updates or warnings, and redoing the design to suit your inclinations.

3. Catch All Errands and Cutoff times: Make a point to catch all undertakings and cutoff times in your organizer or application, no matter what their size or earnestness. This incorporates both present moment and long haul errands, as well as cutoff times for activities or tasks. This will assist you with having a complete perspective on the entirety of your responsibilities and try not to miss any significant cutoff times.

4. Focus on and Dole out Due Dates: Utilize your organizer or application to focus on errands and appoint due dates. This will assist you with envisioning which undertakings are generally significant and should be finished first. You can utilize variety coding, labels, or different elements given by the apparatus to handily distinguish high-need errands.

5. Prepare: Put away customary opportunities to prepare utilizing your

organizer or application. This might include auditing your impending errands, cutoff times, and responsibilities, and apportioning time for explicit undertakings or activities. Preparing can assist you with remaining coordinated and guarantee that you are gaining ground towards your objectives.

6. Audit and Update Consistently: Survey and update your organizer or application routinely to guarantee that it stays modern and mirrors your ongoing needs. This might include check off work, rescheduling or re-focusing on errands on a case by case basis, and adding new undertakings or cutoff times that emerge.

7. Use Updates and Notices: Exploit updates and notices presented by your organizer or application to keep you on target with your undertakings and cutoff times. Set up updates for significant cutoff times, gatherings, or arrangements, and redo the notices to suit your inclinations.

8. Keep it Straightforward: Stay away from overcomplicating your organizer or application with such a large number of classes, labels, or elements that might become overpowering. Keep it straightforward and instinctive, so you can undoubtedly explore and utilize it consistently without feeling overpowered.

9. Practice it regularly: Integrate the utilization of your organizer or application into your everyday daily schedule until it turns into a propensity. Make it a piece of your customary work process to catch, focus on, and track your undertakings and objectives. Consistency is critical to successful association.

10. Be Adaptable: adjust and change your organizer or application framework depending on the situation. Your needs, undertakings, and cutoff times might change over the long haul, so be available to make updates and upgrades to your hierarchical framework as you come.

Dealing with procrastination

Managing stalling can be testing, however here are a few methodologies to assist you with conquering this normal issue:

1. Distinguish the Underlying driver: Consider the reason why you are lingering. Is it because of dread of disappointment, absence of inspiration, overpower, or other basic reasons? Recognizing the main driver of your dawdling can assist you with resolving the fundamental issue and foster procedures to beat it.

2. Break Errands into More modest, Reasonable Advances: Enormous assignments or activities can be overpowering and lead to stalling. Separate them into more modest, more sensible advances, and spotlight them mindfully. This can cause the assignment to feel more feasible and assist you with beginning.

3. Put forth Unambiguous and Reasonable Objectives: Set explicit, quantifiable, and practical objectives for each

undertaking or venture. This can assist you with keeping on track and persuaded, and give a reasonable internal compass. Try not to lay out excessively aggressive objectives that might prompt stalling because of seen trouble or impossibility.

4. Use Time Usage Strategies: Time usage methods, like the Pomodoro Strategy (working in centered eruptions of time followed by brief breaks), can assist you with keeping on track and useful. Set a clock for a particular measure of time and work on the errand without interruptions during that time. Then have some time off prior to continuing the following explosion of centered work.

5. Find Your Efficiency Zone: Focus on your normal rhythms and find your efficiency zone. Certain individuals work best toward the beginning of the day, while others are more useful at night. Recognize the hour of day when you are generally engaged and invigorated, and plan your most significant assignments during that time.

6. Kill Interruptions: Recognize and wipe out or limit interruptions that might be adding to your tarrying. This might include switching off notices on your telephone, shutting pointless tabs on your PC, or tracking down a tranquil and favorable climate for work.

7. Utilize Uplifting feedback: Award yourself subsequent to following through with jobs or gaining ground towards your objectives. This can be basically as straightforward as enjoying some time off, indulging yourself with a little extravagance, or accomplishing something you appreciate. Encouraging feedback can assist you with remaining propelled and make errands more charming.

8. Practice Self-Empathy: Be thoughtful to yourself and practice self-sympathy. Stay away from self-analysis or negative self-talk, as this can additionally fuel stalling. All things considered, recognize that everybody has snapshots of hesitation and be delicate with yourself when you goof. Center around the

headway you make as opposed
flawlessly.

9. Look for Responsibility: Offer your
    objectives and progress with a confided
    in a companion, guide, or partner who
    can consider you responsible. Having
    somebody to check in with or give
    support can assist you with keeping
    focused and defeating delays.

10. Begin: At times, the hardest part is
    absolutely getting everything rolling.
    Beat the desire to postpone or keep away
    from errands by making the principal
    little stride, regardless of how little.
    When you start, you might find it more
    straightforward to gather speed and
    keep chipping away at the errand.

CHAPTER 5

Developing Healthy Eating Habits

Understanding the impact of nutrition on ADHD symptoms

Sustenance can assume a critical part in overseeing side effects of consideration deficiency hyperactivity jumble (ADHD). While there is no particular ADHD diet, research recommends that specific dietary changes might assist with decreasing ADHD side effects in certain people. Here are a few contemplations for grasping the effect of nourishment on ADHD side effects:

1. Adjusted Diet: Eating a reasonable eating regimen that incorporates different entire food sources, like organic products, vegetables, entire grains, lean proteins, and solid fats, can uphold in general cerebrum wellbeing and may assist with overseeing ADHD side effects. Staying away from inordinate admission of handled food

sources, added sugars, and fake added substances is additionally suggested.

2. Protein: Remembering adequate protein for feasts and tidbits can assist with balancing out glucose levels and further develop concentration and fixation. Great wellsprings of protein incorporate lean meats, fish, eggs, dairy or dairy options, beans, nuts, and seeds.

3. Omega-3 Unsaturated fats: Omega-3 unsaturated fats, especially EPA and DHA, found in greasy fish like salmon, mackerel, and sardines, as well as in flaxseeds and chia seeds, have been displayed to have expected benefits for cerebrum wellbeing and may assist with lessening ADHD side effects.

4. Nutrients and Minerals: Satisfactory admission of nutrients and minerals, including iron, zinc, magnesium, and vitamin D, may uphold cerebrum wellbeing and possibly assist with overseeing ADHD side effects. These supplements can be gotten through an even eating regimen or through supplements, if necessary.

5. Food Responsive qualities: A few people with ADHD might have responsive qualities or sensitivity to specific food varieties, like gluten, dairy, or counterfeit added substances. Recognizing and taking out these trigger food varieties from the eating regimen might assist with lessening ADHD side effects at times. Working with a medical care proficient or an enrolled dietitian can help in recognizing food responsive qualities and making a fitting sustenance plan.

6. Caffeine and Sugar: Caffeine and high-sugar food varieties might possibly demolish ADHD side effects in certain people. Restricting the utilization of stimulated refreshments, sweet food varieties, and beverages might assist with overseeing side effects and advance better concentration and conduct.

7. Dinner Arranging and Customary Eating Examples: Laying out normal feast and tidbit times over the course of the day can assist with balancing out glucose levels and forestall energy crashes,

which might influence ADHD side effects. Abstaining from skipping dinners and keeping up with steady eating examples can assist with supporting in general mind wellbeing.

Incorporating a balanced diet into daily routine

Integrating a reasonable eating regimen into your day to day schedule can be gainful for in general wellbeing and prosperity, including overseeing ADHD side effects. Here are a few techniques for integrating a fair eating regimen into your day to day daily schedule:

1. Dinner Arranging: Plan your feasts ahead of time to guarantee that you have various food sources that meet the models of a reasonable eating routine. This can assist you with pursuing better food decisions and try not to hastily go after less nutritious choices.

2. Shopping for food: Make a shopping list in light of your feast plan and stick to it

when you go shopping for food. Abstain from shopping when you're ravenous, as it can prompt motivation acquisition of undesirable food varieties.

3. Breakfast: Begin your day with a nutritious breakfast that incorporates a decent wellspring of protein, solid fats, and entire grains. This can assist with giving supported energy over the course of the day and backing mental capability.

4. Incorporate Various Food sources: Plan to incorporate various food varieties from various nutrition types in your dinners and tidbits. This can assist with guaranteeing that you're getting many supplements required for generally speaking wellbeing and mind capability.

5. Segment Control: Focus on segment sizes to abstain from gorging. Utilize more modest plates and bowls to assist with segment control and stay away from careless eating.

6. Eat Carefully: Practice careful eating by focusing on the taste, surface, and smell

of your food, and eating gradually. Stay away from interruptions, for example, screens or eating in a hurry, and pay attention to your body's craving and completion signals.

7. Hydration: Drink a lot of water over the course of the day to remain hydrated. Water is fundamental for general wellbeing, including cerebrum capability.

8. Nibble Savvy: Pick solid bites that are wealthy in supplements, like new natural products, vegetables, nuts, seeds, yogurt, or hummus, rather than sweet or handled snacks.

9. Limit Handled Food sources: Handled food varieties, high in added sugars, undesirable fats, and counterfeit added substances, ought to be restricted in your eating routine. Pick entire, insignificantly handled food varieties whenever the situation allows.

10. Look for Proficient Direction: On the off chance that you have explicit dietary necessities or limitations, or on the

other hand assuming you're uncertain about how to make a reasonable eating regimen, consider looking for direction from an enlisted dietitian or medical services proficient who can give customized suggestions.

Avoiding triggers such as sugary foods

Staying away from triggers, for example, sweet food sources can be a significant technique in overseeing ADHD side effects. Here are a few ways to keep away from sweet food varieties in your everyday daily schedule:

1. Be aware of added sugars: Focus on food names and fixing records to distinguish added sugars in handled food varieties and refreshments. Added sugars can be masked under different names, for example, sucrose, high-fructose corn syrup, dextrose, and maltose, so getting to know these terms is significant.

2. Pick entire, normal food varieties: Pick entire, regular food varieties whenever the situation allows, as they are commonly lower in added sugars contrasted with handled food sources. Settle on new natural products, vegetables, entire grains, lean proteins, and solid fats, which can give fundamental supplements without the additional sugars.

3. Plan adjusted feasts and bites: Plan adjusted dinners and tidbits that incorporate a mix of protein, solid fats, and complex carbs. This can assist with balancing out glucose levels and lessen desires for sweet food varieties.

4. Stay away from sweet refreshments: Sweet refreshments, for example, pop, natural product juice, caffeinated drinks, and improved teas can be critical wellsprings of added sugars. Select water, natural tea, or unsweetened refreshments all things being equal, and cut off your utilization of sweet beverages.

5. Plan dinners at home: Preparing feasts at home permits you to have command over the fixings and part measures, decreasing the probability of consuming inordinate added sugars. Explore different avenues regarding solid and delightful recipes that consolidate entire, normal food sources.

6. Have sound tidbits close by: Keep solid snacks promptly accessible, like new natural products, vegetables, nuts, seeds, yogurt, or hummus, to fulfill desires and try not to go after sweet food varieties.

7. Practice careful eating: Focus on your body's craving and completion prompts, and practice careful eating to stay away from thoughtless nibbling on sweet food sources. Take as much time as necessary while eating, relish each nibble, and pay attention to your body's signs of appetite and completion.

8. Track down better other options: Search for better options in contrast to sweet food varieties, for example, new natural products, regular sugars like honey or

maple syrup with some restraint, and dim chocolate with higher cocoa content. Try different things with various flavors and surfaces to track down fulfilling options in contrast to sweet food sources.

9. Get support from others: Look for help from family, companions, or a medical care proficient to consider yourself responsible and remain propelled in keeping away from triggers like sweet food varieties. They can give consolation, share tips, and assist you with keeping focused with your dietary objectives.

10. Be aware of close to home eating: Numerous people with ADHD might battle with profound eating, which can include going to sweet food varieties for solace or stress help. Be aware of close to home eating triggers and foster elective survival methods, like activity, reflection, or conversing with a confided in companion or specialist.

Making healthy food choices for better brain health

Pursuing quality food decisions for better mind wellbeing can essentially affect mental capability, including overseeing ADHD side effects. Here are a few explicit ways to integrate mind quality food sources into your eating routine:

1. Eat different brilliant foods grown from the ground: Products of the soil are plentiful in fundamental nutrients, minerals, and cell reinforcements that help mind wellbeing. Expect to remember a beautiful combination of foods grown from the ground for your eating regimen, for example, salad greens, berries, citrus natural products, cruciferous vegetables, and bright ringer peppers.

2. Incorporate entire grains: Entire grains, like earthy colored rice, quinoa, oats, and entire grain bread, are wealthy in fiber and give supported energy to the mind. They additionally contain significant supplements like B nutrients

that are fundamental for mental capability.

3. Pick lean proteins: Lean proteins, like poultry, fish, beans, lentils, tofu, and Greek yogurt, give significant amino acids that are important for synapse creation, which influences state of mind, fixation, and concentration.

4. Consolidate solid fats: Sound fats, like those tracked down in nuts, seeds, avocados, greasy fish (e.g., salmon, fish, mackerel), and olive oil, are significant for cerebrum wellbeing. They give fundamental omega-3 unsaturated fats that help mental capability and assist with diminishing aggravation in the mind.

5. Limit added sugars: High admission of added sugars can adversely affect mental capability and worsen ADHD side effects. Stay away from or limit food varieties and refreshments that are high in added sugars, like sweet bites, pastries, pop, and improved drinks.

6. Remain hydrated: Drying out can hinder mental capability, so it's essential to remain appropriately hydrated. Drink a lot of water over the course of the day to help ideal mind wellbeing.

7. Think about cancer prevention agents: Cell reinforcement rich food varieties, like blueberries, strawberries, spinach, kale, and dim chocolate, have been displayed to have neuroprotective properties and may uphold cerebrum wellbeing.

8. Limit handled food sources: Handled food sources are much of the time high in unfortunate fats, sodium, and added sugars, and may adversely affect mental capability. Limit your admission of handled food varieties and select entire, negligibly handled food sources whenever the situation allows.

9. Practice careful eating: Focus on your dietary patterns and practice careful eating. Abstain from eating thoughtlessly, and set aside some margin to relish each nibble, partaking

in the flavors, surfaces, and fragrances
of your food.

10. Look for proficient direction: In the
event that you have explicit dietary
necessities or concerns, consider talking
with an enlisted dietitian or medical care
proficient for customized direction on
settling on good food decisions to help
mind wellbeing.

CHAPTER 6

Practicing Stress Management Techniques

Recognizing and managing stress triggers

Perceiving and overseeing pressure triggers is a significant part of overseeing ADHD side effects and keeping up with in general mental prosperity. Here are a few techniques to help you distinguish and oversee pressure triggers:

1. Mindfulness: Focus on your viewpoints, sentiments, and ways of behaving to recognize designs that might set off pressure. Notice circumstances, individuals, or occasions that will generally build your feelings of anxiety. Keeping a diary or utilizing a pressure following application can assist you with recognizing normal pressure triggers.

2. Recognize stressors: Make a rundown of the particular circumstances, individuals, or occasions that trigger pressure for you. Be basically as unambiguous as conceivable in

distinguishing these triggers, and attempt to pinpoint the fundamental justifications for why they cause pressure.

3. Prepare: Whenever you have recognized your pressure triggers, foster an arrangement to proactively oversee them. For instance, assuming you realize that cutoff times at work will quite often set off pressure, prepare by breaking errands into more modest, sensible advances, setting reasonable cutoff times, and designating time for taking care of oneself.

4. Practice pressure decreasing strategies: Integrate pressure lessening procedures into your everyday daily schedule. This might incorporate care reflection, profound breathing activities, moderate muscle unwinding, yoga, or other unwinding strategies that work for you. These procedures can assist you with overseeing pressure when triggers emerge.

5. Put down sound stopping points: Figure out how to define solid limits to

safeguard yourself from superfluous pressure. This might include saying "no" as needs be, appointing errands, and focusing on taking care of oneself. Defining limits can assist you with overseeing pressure triggers connected with overcommitment or feeling overpowered.

6. Construct an emotionally supportive network: Encircle yourself with steady individuals who can give you constant reassurance and useful help. This might incorporate relatives, companions, or a specialist. Having an emotionally supportive network set up can assist you with overseeing pressure triggers by giving an outlet to venting, critical thinking, and getting a viewpoint.

7. Practice using time productively: Unfortunately using time productively can be a critical pressure trigger for some people with ADHD. Carry out methodologies, for example, making plans for the day, focusing on undertakings, and utilizing time usage instruments, for example, schedules or efficiency applications, to all the more

likely deal with your time and decrease pressure.

8. Practice taking care of oneself: Dealing with your physical and mental prosperity is fundamental in overseeing pressure triggers. Try to get sufficient rest, eat a fair eating routine, take part in normal actual activity, and practice self-empathy. Dealing with yourself can assist you with better overseeing pressure triggers and constructing strength.

9. Look for proficient assistance: On the off chance that pressure triggers are overpowering and influencing your everyday existence, think about looking for proficient assistance from a specialist or instructor. They can give you instruments and strategies to more readily oversee pressure, and proposition backing and direction custom-made to your singular requirements.

Incorporating relaxation techniques into daily routine

Integrating unwinding strategies into your everyday schedule can be exceptionally useful for overseeing pressure, working on mental prosperity, and lessening ADHD side effects. Here are a few methodologies to assist you with incorporating unwinding strategies into your everyday daily practice:

1. Plan unwinding time: Very much like you plan time for different exercises in your day, put away unambiguous time for unwinding. This can be as committed breaks during the day or assigned unwinding periods in the first part of the day or night. Treat this time as non-debatable and focus on it in your timetable.

2. Pick unwinding strategies that work for you: There are different unwinding methods accessible, like care reflection, profound breathing activities, moderate muscle unwinding, directed symbolism, or body filter. Try different things with various procedures and pick the ones that turn out best for yourself as well as your necessities. You may likewise join

various strategies or alter them to suit your inclinations.

3. Establish a loosening up climate: Find a tranquil and agreeable space where you can rehearse unwinding methods without interruptions. This can be an assigned unwinding corner in your home, a recreation area, or some other tranquil area. Think about utilizing props like an agreeable seat, pads, or delicate lighting to establish a relieving climate.

4. Begin little and be steady: It's vital to begin little and be reliable with your unwinding practice. Start with more limited meetings and progressively increment the span over the long run. Consistency is critical, so plan to rehearse unwinding strategies everyday or as often as conceivable to receive the greatest rewards.

5. Coordinate unwinding into everyday exercises: You can likewise integrate unwinding methods into your day to day exercises. For instance, you can rehearse profound breathing activities while

holding up in line, do a speedy body examination throughout a break, or practice care while eating or strolling. This can assist you with incorporating unwinding into your day to day daily practice without expecting to save committed time for it.

6. Use unwinding methods as adapting devices: notwithstanding booked unwinding time, you can likewise involve unwinding strategies as adapting apparatuses during seasons of pressure or overpower. At the point when you notice pressure or ADHD side effects rising, take a couple of seconds to rehearse unwinding methods to assist with quieting your psyche and body.

7. Make it pleasant: Unwinding strategies ought to be charming and not feel like a task. Track down ways of making it pleasurable, like utilizing loosening up fragrances, paying attention to quieting music, or consolidating exercises you appreciate, as delicate yoga or a nature stroll, into your unwinding schedule. This can assist you with anticipating your unwinding practice and make it a

positive piece of your everyday daily schedule.

Practicing mindfulness and meditation

Rehearsing care and contemplation can be powerful techniques for overseeing pressure, further developing concentration, and diminishing ADHD side effects. Here are a few ways to integrate care and reflection into your everyday daily practice:

1. Begin with short meetings: In the event that you are new to care and reflection, it's ideal to begin with more limited meetings and continuously increment the span as you become more agreeable. Start with only a couple of moments of care or reflection practice each day and step by step move gradually up to longer meetings.

2. Track down a calm and agreeable space: Pick a peaceful and agreeable space where you can rehearse care or contemplation without interruptions. This can be an assigned spot in your

home, a recreation area, or some other quiet area. Think about utilizing props, for example, a pad or an agreeable seat to help your stance during contemplation.

3. Follow directed contemplations: Directed reflections are a superb method for beginning your care and contemplation practice. You can find various directed contemplation assets on the web, for example, applications, sites, or recordings. Directed contemplations give bit by bit guidelines and assist you with keeping on track during your training.

4. Practice care in everyday exercises: Care can be rehearsed in different exercises over the course of your day. For instance, you can rehearse careful eating by focusing on the taste, surface, and smell of your food, or practice careful strolling by focusing on your strides and the sensations in your body as you walk. Incorporating care into your everyday exercises can assist you with carrying more attention to the current second and develop a feeling of quiet.

5. Try different things with various
    strategies: There are different care and
    contemplation procedures, for example,
    body check, breath mindfulness, adoring
    graciousness reflection, and some more.
    Explore different avenues regarding
    various procedures and find what turns
    out best for you. You can likewise
    consolidate various methods or alter
    them to suit your inclinations.

6. Be non-critical and patient: Care and
    contemplation are rehearses that require
    tolerance and non-critical mindfulness.
    Be caring to yourself and try not to pass
    judgment on your viewpoints, feelings,
    or encounters during your training.
    Basically notice them with interest and
    without judgment, and delicately take
    your concentration back to your picked
    point of concentration, like your breath
    or body sensations.

7. Regularly practice it: Consistency is key
    with regards to care and contemplation.
    Attempt to make it a day to day
    propensity by saving committed time for
    training, regardless of whether it's only a

couple of moments each day. Consider coordinating care and contemplation into your morning or night schedule to assist you with laying out a predictable practice.

8. Be adaptable and versatile: Care and reflection practices may not generally go as expected, and that is not a problem. Be adaptable and versatile, and don't get deterred in the event that your psyche meanders or on the other hand assuming you find it trying to remain on track. It's a typical piece of the training, and with time and consistency, you'll probably see enhancements.

Engaging in activities to reduce stress and anxiety

Taking part in exercises to diminish pressure and uneasiness can be gainful for overseeing ADHD side effects. Here are a few techniques for integrating pressure diminishing exercises into your everyday daily practice:

1. Work out: Actual activity has been demonstrated to be a viable pressure

minimizer. Standard active work, like
strolling, running, swimming, or
participating in different types of
vigorous activity, can assist with
delivering endorphins, which are normal
temperaments lifting synthetic
compounds in the mind. Go for the gold
30 minutes of moderate-power practice
most days of the week to assist with
lessening pressure and nervousness.

2. Care and contemplation: As examined
    prior, rehearsing care and reflection can
    assist with quieting the brain, diminish
    pressure, and further develop center.
    You can integrate short care or
    contemplation meetings into your
    everyday daily schedule to help you
    unwind and oversee pressure. There are
    different care and contemplation
    procedures accessible, so find the ones
    that turn out best for you.

3. Leisure activities and imaginative
    exercises: Taking part in side interests
    or imaginative exercises that you
    appreciate can be a compelling method
    for lessening pressure and tension.
    Whether it's painting, playing an

instrument, cooking, planting, or whatever other action that gives you pleasure, set aside a few minutes for it in your day to day everyday practice to help you unwind and loosen up.

4. Social associations: Investing energy with strong loved ones, or participating in friendly exercises that you appreciate, can assist with decreasing pressure and tension. Interfacing with others, sharing encounters, and getting basic reassurance can be advantageous for overseeing pressure and further developing your general prosperity.

5. Time in nature: Investing energy in nature, for example, taking a stroll in the park, climbing, or essentially sitting in a quiet regular setting, can assist with lessening pressure and tension. Nature meaningfully affects the brain and body, and being encircled by regular magnificence can help you unwind and revive.

6. Breathing activities: Profound breathing activities can assist with quieting the sensory system and lessen pressure and

tension. You can rehearse basic breathing activities, for example, stomach breathing or box breathing, at whatever point you feel worried or restless to help you unwind and recapture the center.

7. Using time effectively: Successful using time productively can assist with diminishing pressure and tension by assisting you with remaining coordinated and on top of undertakings. Prepare, focus on errands, and separate them into more modest sensible advances. Use apparatuses like schedules, daily agendas, or efficiency applications to assist you with remaining coordinated and decrease pressure connected with time pressure.

8. Taking care of oneself: Dealing with yourself is urgent for overseeing pressure and tension. Make a point to focus on taking care of oneself exercises like getting sufficient rest, eating a decent eating routine, and rehearsing great cleanliness. Dealing with your physical and mental prosperity can assist you with better overseeing

pressure and tension in your regular routine.

CHAPTER 7

Building Social Skills and Relationships

Developing healthy communication skills

Creating solid relational abilities can be valuable for overseeing ADHD side effects and further developing associations with others. Here are a few techniques for creating sound relational abilities:

1. Undivided attention: Practice undivided attention, which includes completely zeroing in on the speaker, staying away from interference, and showing compassion and understanding. Rehash or rework what the speaker said to guarantee you have perceived their message accurately. Stay away from interruptions, for example, really looking at your telephone or different assignments, while somebody is addressing you.

2. Explanation: In the event that you're uncertain about something, make it a point to request explanation. It's smarter to request explanation than to make presumptions or get the message wrong. Posing inquiries can likewise show your advantage and commitment to the discussion.

3. Emphaticness: Practice confident correspondence, which includes offering your viewpoints, sentiments, and requirements in a reasonable and deferential way. Keep away from detached correspondence, which might include trying not to struggle or put yourself out there in a bashful or regretful way, and forceful correspondence, which might include being fierce, impolite, or discourteous. Decisive correspondence can assist you with articulating your thoughts really without being excessively inactive or forceful.

4. Profound guideline: Dealing with your feelings and answering others in a cool headed way is a significant part of sound correspondence. Practice methods for

close to home guidelines, like taking full breaths, building up to ten, or having some time off when you feel yourself becoming overpowered or profound during a discussion. This can assist you with staying cool headed and convey in a more successful way.

5. Sympathy: Show compassion towards others by attempting to figure out their point of view, feelings, and necessities. Recognize and approve their sentiments and encounters, regardless of whether you may not concur with them. This can assist fabricate trust and compatibility in your associations with others.

6. Non-verbal correspondence: Focus on non-verbal signs, like non-verbal communication, looks, and manner of speaking. These signals can give significant data about how the other individual is feeling and what they are attempting to convey. Likewise, be aware of your own non-verbal signals and guarantee they line up with your expected message.

7. Compromise: Foster abilities for settling clashes in a helpful and solid way. Trying not to clash or allow them to raise can adversely influence connections and correspondence. Practice strategies for viable compromise, like utilizing "I" articulations to communicate your sentiments, effectively paying attention to the next individual's viewpoint, and tracking down commonly adequate arrangements.

8. Adaptability: Be available to input, alternate points of view, and valuable analysis. Try not to be cautious or cavalier, and endeavor to figure out some mutual interest and that's employers of all interested parties. Adaptability in correspondence can assist you with exploring troublesome discussions and construct sound connections.

9. Practice, practice, practice: Relational abilities are created over the long run with training. Show restraint toward yourself and continue to rehearse your relational abilities in various settings

and with various individuals. Ponder your correspondence style and persistently work on further developing it.

Managing social interaction and Relationships

Overseeing social connections and connections can be trying for people with ADHD, however it is feasible to foster successful procedures for exploring social circumstances. Here are a few ways to oversee social connections and connections:

1. Foster mindfulness: Figuring out your own ADHD side effects, triggers, and difficulties in friendly corporations can assist you with better overseeing them. Think about your assets and shortcomings in friendly circumstances, and be aware of what your ADHD side effects might mean for your correspondence, conduct, and associations with others.

2. Practice undivided attention: Effectively pay attention to others in friendly collaborations, which includes offering

them your full consideration, staying away from interference, and showing veritable interest in what they are talking about. Try not to hinder or get diverted by different things while somebody is addressing you.

3. Utilize viewable signs: Utilize obvious prompts, for example, keeping in touch, gesturing, and utilizing suitable looks, to show that you are participating in the discussion and effectively tuning in. These viewable signs can assist you with better associating with others and show that you are keen on what they need to say.

4. Foster sympathy: Practice compassion towards others by attempting to grasp their viewpoint, feelings, and necessities. Show empathy and understanding towards their sentiments and encounters, regardless of whether you may not completely concur with them. Sympathy can assist assembling more grounded associations and associations with others.

5. Foster interactive abilities: Work on creating interactive abilities, for example, starting discussions, keeping up with suitable individual space, utilizing fitting manner of speaking, and figuring out expressive gestures. Think about looking for help from a specialist, guide, or interactive abilities gathering to work on your interactive abilities and gain trust in friendly collaborations.

6. Put down clear stopping points: Laying out and keeping up with clear limits in connections is significant for overseeing social communications. Be emphatic in communicating your own necessities, inclinations, and impediments, and impart them plainly and differentially to other people. This can assist with keeping away from misconceptions and clashes in connections.

7. Oversee impulsivity: Impulsivity is a typical side effect of ADHD that can influence social collaborations. Practice drive control procedures, like taking full breaths, building up to ten, or pausing for a minute to think prior to answering or making a move in friendly

circumstances. This can assist you with keeping away from imprudent responses that may adversely influence connections.

8. Foster social help: Encircle yourself with a strong informal organization of understanding and tolerating people who know about your ADHD and offer help. Having an emotionally supportive network can assist you with overseeing social difficulties and offer profound help in troublesome social circumstances.

9. Practice social critical thinking: Foster critical thinking abilities for social circumstances, like settling clashes, overseeing mistaken assumptions, and tracking down commonly satisfactory arrangements. Ponder past friendly communications and gain from them to further develop your social critical thinking abilities.

10. Practice self-sympathy: Be thoughtful and sympathetic towards yourself in friendly associations. Recognize that you might have difficulties because of ADHD

yet additionally perceive your assets and progress. Keep away from self-fault or negative self-talk, and practice self-empathy in overseeing social communications and connections.

Dealing with social challenges related to ADHD

Social difficulties connected with ADHD can be baffling and influence different parts of day to day existence, including connections, work, and in general prosperity. Here are a few systems for managing social difficulties connected with ADHD:

1. Teach yourself as well as other people: Find out about ADHD and its effect on friendly corporations. Teach yourself about the side effects, difficulties, and procedures for overseeing ADHD in friendly circumstances. Share this data with dear companions, family, and other significant people in your day to day existence to assist them with better figuring out your condition.

2. Practice mindfulness: Foster mindfulness of your ADHD side effects and what they might mean for your social communications. Think about your assets and shortcomings in friendly circumstances, and be aware of any hasty or hyperactive ways of behaving that might influence your associations with others.

3. Use ADHD-accommodating methodologies: Use ADHD-accommodating techniques, like obvious signals, updates, and clocks, to assist you with remaining on track, coordinated, and deal with your time successfully in friendly circumstances. For instance, utilizing an organizer or an update application on your telephone can assist you with monitoring social responsibilities and stay away from failing to remember significant occasions or arrangements.

4. Foster ways of dealing with especially difficult times: Distinguish and foster survival techniques for overseeing social difficulties connected with ADHD. This might incorporate rehearsing drive

control strategies, overseeing interruptions, utilizing unwinding methods to oversee pressure, and rehearsing successful relational abilities.

5. Look for help: Contact a specialist or advisor who can give direction and backing in overseeing social difficulties connected with ADHD. They can assist you with creating survival techniques, work on interactive abilities, and offer help in exploring social circumstances.

6. Set sensible assumptions: Be practical about your social capacities and try not to contrast yourself with others. Acknowledge that you might have difficulties connected with ADHD and that it's alright to commit errors or have misfortunes in friendly communications. Set practical assumptions for you and others, and be thoughtful to yourself all the while.

7. Convey straightforwardly: Discuss transparently with dear companions, family, and other significant people in your day to day existence about your difficulties connected with ADHD.

Speak the truth about your battles, constraints, and requirements in friendly circumstances. Open correspondence can help other people comprehend and uphold you better.

8. Practice interactive abilities: Work on creating interactive abilities through training and openness to social circumstances. Work on starting discussions, keeping in touch, utilizing a fitting manner of speaking, and figuring out expressive gestures. Consider looking for help from a specialist or partaking in an interactive abilities gathering to additionally foster your interactive abilities.

9. Fabricate a steady interpersonal organization: Encircle yourself with a strong informal community of understanding and tolerating people who can offer close to home help, understanding, and acknowledgment of your ADHD-related social difficulties. Building major areas of strength for a framework can assist you with overseeing social difficulties and further develop your general prosperity.

10. Practice taking care of oneself: Deal with
yourself genuinely, inwardly, and
intellectually. Practice taking care of
oneself procedures, like getting
sufficient rest, eating great, participating
in customary actual activity, and
overseeing pressure through unwinding
strategies or care. Dealing with yourself
can assist you with better overseeing
social difficulties connected with ADHD.

Building a support system

Building an emotionally supportive network
can be a fundamental piece of overseeing
ADHD really. Having a steady organization of
people who comprehend and acknowledge your
demands connected with ADHD can offer close
to home help, useful help, and support. Here
are a few procedures for building an
emotionally supportive network:

1. Recognize steady people: Distinguish
    individuals in your day to day existence
    who are understanding, non-critical,
    and acknowledging of your ADHD

demands. This might incorporate dear companions, relatives, accomplices, associates, or guides. Search for people who will tune in, offer help, and give consolation without condemning.

2. Instruct your emotionally supportive network: Teach your emotionally supportive network about ADHD, its side effects, difficulties, and effect on your life. Share data about your encounters with ADHD, including what it means for your day to day routine, work, connections, and generally prosperity. This can assist them with better figuring out your condition and offer suitable help.

3. Impart straightforwardly: Be transparent with your emotionally supportive network about your ADHD difficulties, requirements, and impediments. Convey transparently about your battles, triumphs, and any help you might require. Request help when required and convey your sentiments and concerns.

4. Join support gatherings: Consider joining support gatherings or online networks explicitly for people with ADHD. These gatherings can give a steady local area where you can interface with other people who have comparable encounters and difficulties. You can share encounters, trade survival methods, and gain from other people who comprehend what you're going through.

5. Look for proficient help: Think about looking for proficient help from a specialist, guide, or mentor who has insight in working with people with ADHD. An expert can give direction, survival methods, and daily reassurance custom-made to your novel necessities and difficulties.

6. Take part in ADHD-related occasions: Go to occasions, studios, or workshops connected with ADHD. These occasions can give potential chances to interface with other people who have ADHD, gain from specialists, and gain bits of knowledge and procedures for overseeing ADHD actually.

7. Fabricate a help group: Collect a group of experts who can uphold you in overseeing ADHD. This might incorporate a specialist, guide, therapist, mentor, or other medical services experts who spend significant time in ADHD. Team up with them to foster techniques and instruments for overseeing ADHD challenges actually.

8. Cultivate solid connections: Sustain sound associations with strong people who comprehend and acknowledge your ADHD demands. Encircle yourself with individuals who elevate you, empower your assets, and back your objectives. Limit communications with people who are critical, unsupportive, or cavalier of your ADHD challenges.

9. Practice self-promotion: Promoter for yourself by obviously communicating your necessities, limits, and assumptions to your emotionally supportive network. Be self-assured in conveying your expectation to successfully deal with your ADHD

challenges, and attest your privileges in getting proper help and facilities.

10. Be a steady individual from others' emotionally supportive networks: Building an emotionally supportive network is a two-way road. Offer help, understanding, and consolation to others in your emotionally supportive network who may likewise be managing difficulties. Offer compassion, approval, and pragmatic help to other people, similarly as you might want to get from them.

CHAPTER 8

Balancing Screen Time and Digital Wellness

Understanding the impact of excessive screen time on ADHD side effects

Unnecessary screen time, including delayed utilization of electronic gadgets, for example, cell phones, tablets, PCs, and TVs, might possibly affect ADHD side effects adversely. Here are a few contemplations in regards to the effect of unreasonable screen time on ADHD side effects:

1. Expanded interruption: Investing unreasonable energy in screens can prompt expanded interruption and trouble in centering, which are now normal difficulties for people with ADHD. The consistent boosts and notices from screens can additionally disturb focus and obstruct efficiency.

2. Diminished actual work: Inordinate screen time can prompt an inactive way

of life, which can adversely influence actual wellbeing and intensify ADHD side effects. Absence of actual work can prompt expanded anxiety, impulsivity, and hyperactivity, which are normal side effects of ADHD.

3. Rest interruptions: Screen time, particularly before sleep time, can impede rest quality and amount. Unfortunate rest can fuel ADHD side effects, including obliviousness, impulsivity, and hyperactivity, and can influence generally mental and profound working.

4. Expanded impulsivity and hazard taking ways of behaving: Investing unreasonable energy in screens, particularly via online entertainment, can prompt rash and chance taking ways of behaving. This can bring about diminished self-guideline and expanded incautious independent direction, which can adversely influence ADHD side effects and in general working.

5. Decreased social communications: Investing unreasonable energy in

screens can prompt diminished up close and personal social collaborations, which are significant for building and keeping up with interactive abilities, connections, and profound prosperity. Diminished social connections can affect interactive abilities improvement and fuel social difficulties frequently connected with ADHD.

6. Blue light openness: The blue light radiated by screens can affect rest quality and disturb circadian rhythms, possibly fueling ADHD side effects. Blue light openness at night can upset the creation of melatonin, a chemical that manages rest, prompting rest unsettling influences and deteriorating ADHD side effects.

7. Expanded hazard of habit: Inordinate screen time, particularly with specific sorts of content or exercises, can build the gamble of fixation or tricky use, prompting impulsive ways of behaving and further fueling ADHD side effects.

8.

    a. It's vital to perceive that unreasonable screen time might possibly affect ADHD side effects adversely. To oversee screen time successfully, think about the accompanying methodologies:

9. Put down certain boundaries: Lay out clear limits and cutoff points on screen time, both with regards to length and sorts of exercises. Consider utilizing screen using time productively applications, clocks, or setting explicit time windows for screen use to stay away from inordinate and uncontrolled screen time.

10. Focus on actual work and outside time: Make a point to integrate customary active work and open air time into your daily schedule. Actual work can assist with overseeing ADHD side effects, further develop temperament, and lessen stationary ways of behaving related to inordinate screen time.

11. Make innovation free zones: Lay out assigned innovation free zones in your home, like the room or during feasts, to advance sound propensities and decrease over the top screen time.

12. Practice great rest cleanliness: Make a
    sleep time schedule that incorporates
    limiting screen time before rest,
    decreasing blue light openness, and
    advancing great rest cleanliness
    rehearses, for example, laying out a
    normal rest plan and making a
    loosening up sleep time schedule.

13. Cultivate up close and personal social
    connections: Really try to take part in
    eye to eye social communications, like
    investing energy with loved ones, taking
    part in leisure activities, or joining
    gatherings. This can assist with
    decreasing inordinate screen time and
    advance solid social connections, which
    are significant for overseeing ADHD side
    effects.

14. Be aware of content and exercises: Be
    aware of the substance and exercises you
    participate in on screens. Try not to
    participate in exercises that might be
    habit-forming or excessively animating,
    and focus on exercises that are gainful
    for your prosperity, like instructive

substance, unwinding strategies, or care works out.

15. Look for proficient assistance if necessary: On the off chance that you figure out that extreme screen opportunity is essentially influencing your ADHD side effects and generally speaking prosperity, think about looking for proficient assistance from a specialist.

Setting healthy boundaries with technology

Defining sound limits with innovation is fundamental for overseeing screen time really and advancing in general prosperity. Here are a few ways to define sound limits with innovation:

1. Characterize your needs: Figure out what exercises and assignments are generally essential to you and focus on them over screen time. This can incorporate work, family time, exercise, side interests, and taking care of oneself. By explaining your needs, you can define

limits around innovation to guarantee that it doesn't disrupt your significant exercises.

2. Lay out assigned innovation free times and zones: Make assigned times and zones in your everyday schedule where innovation isn't permitted. For instance, you can set "no innovation" hours before sleep time, during dinners, or during assigned family time. You can likewise lay out innovation free zones in your home, like the room or the feasting region, to make solid propensities and lessen extreme screen time.

3. Set explicit time limits: Decide explicit time limits for various sorts of screen exercises, like web-based entertainment, gaming, or sitting in front of the television, and stick to them. Use screen using time productively applications or inherent highlights on gadgets to set clocks or suggestions to assist you with remaining responsible to your time limits.

4. Practice careful and deliberate innovation use: Be careful and

purposeful about how you use
innovation. Keep away from thoughtless
looking over or unending perusing, and
on second thought, use innovation with
reason and goal. Put forth unambiguous
objectives for your innovation use and
try not to get found out in that frame of
mind of aloof utilization.

5. Take normal innovation breaks:
   Timetable customary innovation breaks
   over the course of your day or week.
   Utilize these breaks to take part in
   different exercises, like activity,
   perusing, or investing energy in nature.
   Enjoying reprieves from screens can
   assist with lessening eye strain, further
   develop act, and advance by and large
   prosperity.

6. Convey and show sound innovation use
   with others: On the off chance that
   you're living with others, impart and lay
   out common arrangements about solid
   innovation use. Energize and show solid
   innovation propensities with your
   family, companions, and partners to
   establish a strong climate for defining
   and keeping up with limits.

7. Be aware of blue light openness: Blue light produced by screens can influence rest quality and upset circadian rhythms. Be aware of your blue light openness, particularly at night, and consider utilizing blue light channels or changing to "night mode" on your gadgets to lessen the effect on your rest.

8. Practice taking care of oneself: Focus on taking care of oneself exercises, like activity, care, and unwinding methods, over exorbitant screen time. Dealing with your physical and mental prosperity can assist you keep up with sound limits with innovation and oversee pressure and ADHD side effects really.

Incorporating screen-free activities into daily routine

Integrating without screen exercises into your everyday schedule can be beneficial for overseeing ADHD side effects, diminishing pressure, further developing concentration, and advancing in general prosperity. Here are a few ways to integrate without screen exercises into your everyday daily practice:

1. Plan and timetable without screen exercises: Very much like you plan and timetable your screen time, focus on it to plan and timetable sans screen exercises also. This can incorporate exercises like activity, perusing, side interests, open air exercises, mingling, or participating in imaginative pursuits. Put these exercises on your schedule or plan for the day to guarantee they are focused on and integrated into your day to day everyday practice.

2. Make a devoted screen-extra energy: Put away a particular time every day or week that is assigned as screen-leisure time. This can be a set opportunity in the first part of the day or night, or an assigned day of the week where you focus on being without screen. Utilize this chance to participate in different exercises that you appreciate and that advance your physical, mental, and close to home prosperity.

3. Track down choices to screen-based exercises: Distinguish exercises that you appreciate and that don't include screens. This can incorporate exercises like activity, journaling, drawing, cooking, planting, playing an instrument, or investing energy in nature. Explore different avenues regarding various exercises and find what impacts you, and integrate them into your everyday daily schedule as sans screen choices.

4. Put down stopping points around screen time: Lay out clear limits around your screen time to make space for without screen exercises. For instance, you can draw certain lines on how much time you spend via web-based entertainment, gaming, or staring at the television, and utilize the additional time for without screen exercises. Use screen using time productively applications or elements on your gadgets to assist you with remaining responsible to your limits.

5. Practice care and presence in non-screen exercises: While taking part in sans screen exercises, practice care and

presence. Be completely present at the time and submerge yourself in the movement without interruptions. This can assist you with completely getting a charge out of and benefit from the sans screen movement, and work on your capacity to concentrate and be available in different parts of your life too.

6. Include others in without screen exercises: Participate in without screen exercises with others, like family, companions, or associates. This can incorporate exercises, for example, tabletop games, outside sports, cooking together, or taking a walk. Including others can make the action more agreeable as well as cultivate social associations and connections.

7. Be adaptable and versatile: Recall that integrating without screen exercises into your everyday schedule is an individual decision, and it's vital to be adaptable and versatile. Every so often might be more occupied than others, and it's OK to change your without screen exercises in light of your timetable and conditions. The key is to find an equilibrium that

works for yourself and supports your general prosperity.

Practicing digital wellness for better mental health

Rehearsing advanced wellbeing is significant for keeping up with better psychological wellbeing, particularly in the present innovation driven world. Here are a few methodologies for integrating computerized wellbeing into your everyday practice:

1. Put down sound stopping points: Lay out clear limits around your computerized gadget use. This can remember drawing certain lines for screen time, keeping away from exorbitant utilization of virtual entertainment, and diminishing pointless advanced interruptions. Make assigned "no-gadget" zones or times in your day, for example, during dinners, before sleep time, or during significant exercises, to consider continuous concentration and unwinding.

2. Practice care: Be aware of your advanced gadget use and its effect on your emotional well-being. Notice how long you spend on screens, how certain computerized exercises cause you to feel, and whether they add to pressure, uneasiness, or other pessimistic feelings. Enjoy reprieves, practice profound breathing or unwinding strategies, and remain present at the time, in any event, while utilizing advanced gadgets.

3. Develop sound web-based propensities: Be deliberate about the substance you consume and the web-based networks you draw in with. Encircle yourself with positive, elevating, and motivating computerized content that advances mental prosperity. Unfollow or quiet records that trigger pessimistic feelings or correlations. Try not to take part in poisonous web-based discussions or ways of behaving that can hurt your psychological well-being.

4. Focus on taking care of oneself: Focus on taking care of oneself in your day to day everyday practice, both on the web and disconnected. Enjoy reprieves from

screens and take part in exercises that advance your emotional well-being, like activity, investing energy in nature, associating with friends and family, rehearsing leisure activities, or taking part in care rehearsals. Make sure to rehearse self-empathy and focus on taking care of oneself as a fundamental piece of your computerized wellbeing schedule.

5. Look for help: Assuming you're battling with emotional well-being issues connected with advanced use, go ahead and support. Converse with a confided in companion, relative, or emotional wellness proficient. They can give you direction, backing, and systems to deal with the effect of advanced use on your psychological wellness.

6. Use innovation to help psychological well-being: While unreasonable computerized use can adversely affect psychological well-being, innovation can likewise be utilized in a positive manner to help psychological wellness. There are various applications and computerized devices accessible that proposition

directed reflection, stress decrease works out, rest following, temperament following, and other emotional wellness assets. Utilize these devices carefully and purposefully to help your psychological prosperity.

7. Practice great rest cleanliness: Appropriate rest is pivotal for emotional well-being. Make a sound rest schedule that includes disengaging from screens no less than one hour before sleep time, keeping your room liberated from computerized interruptions, and pursuing great rest cleanliness routines, for example, keeping a reliable rest plan, making a loosening up sleep time schedule, and guaranteeing an agreeable rest climate.

CHAPTER 9

Coping with Emotional Regulation

Understanding the emotional challenges faced by teens with ADHD

Adolescents with ADHD (Consideration Shortage/Hyperactivity Problem) frequently face novel inner difficulties that can affect their prosperity and day to day working. A portion of the normal personal difficulties looked by youngsters with ADHD might include:

1. Dissatisfaction and outrage: Youngsters with ADHD might battle with dealing with their impulsivity, which can prompt imprudent explosions of disappointment or outrage. They might battle with profound guidelines, finding it challenging to get a grip on their feelings and respond improperly in specific circumstances.

2. Low confidence: Adolescents with ADHD might encounter low confidence because of challenges in gathering scholastic, social, or conduct

assumptions. They might contrast
themselves with their companions and
feel lacking, prompting a negative self-
discernment.

3. Uneasiness and despondency:
   Adolescents with ADHD might be at
   expanded risk for creating nervousness
   and sadness. The difficulties they face in
   dealing with their ADHD side effects,
   like trouble with concentration,
   association, and using time effectively,
   may add to sensations of stress,
   overpower, and disappointment, which
   can fuel tension and sorrow.

4. Dismissal and social troubles: Teenagers
   with ADHD might battle with social
   corporations and face difficulties in
   making and keeping up with fellowships.
   They might experience issues with drive
   control, intruding on others, or perusing
   expressive gestures, which can prompt
   dismissal, social disengagement, and
   hardships in framing significant
   associations with peers.

5. Scholastic battles: Adolescents with
   ADHD might confront difficulties in

scholarly settings, like trouble with association, using time effectively, and finishing tasks. This can prompt disappointment, stress, and hardships in measuring up to scholastic assumptions, which might affect their confidence and generally close to home prosperity.

6. Close to home dysregulation: Youngsters with ADHD might encounter troubles in directing their feelings, which can prompt emotional episodes, peevishness, and impulsivity. They might battle with overseeing extreme feelings, like dissatisfaction, outrage, or bitterness, which can influence their connections and everyday working.

7. Sensations of being overpowered: Youngsters with ADHD might feel overpowered by the requests and assumptions for day to day existence, like school, extracurricular exercises, social associations, and obligations at home. This can prompt sensations of stress, nervousness, and being not able to adapt to the requests put upon them.

Identifying triggers and managing emotions effectively

Recognizing triggers and dealing with feelings really is a significant part of self-guideline, especially for people with ADHD. Here are a few techniques that can help:

1. Mindfulness: Urge people with ADHD to foster mindfulness by focusing on their viewpoints, sentiments, and ways of behaving. Assist them with distinguishing their triggers - circumstances, individuals, or occasions that will generally be major areas of strength for incite reactions. This can incorporate circumstances where they might feel overpowered, baffled, or focused. Whenever triggers are recognized, people can more readily expect and deal with their feelings.

2. Feeling naming: Urge people with ADHD to mark their feelings. This can help them perceive and recognize their feelings, which is the most important phase in overseeing them really. They can utilize words to depict their feelings, for example, "I'm feeling furious," "I'm

feeling restless," or "I'm feeling overpowered." This can assist them with acquiring clearness about their feelings and answer them in a more purposeful manner.

3. Feeling guideline techniques: Train people with ADHD different procedures to control their feelings. This can incorporate profound breathing, moderate muscle unwinding, representation, or other unwinding strategies. Urge them to rehearse these systems when they notice their feelings beginning to raise, and make them a normal piece of their daily practice to foster profound flexibility.

4. Mental rebuilding: Help people with ADHD recognize and challenge pessimistic or pointless considerations that might add to their close to home dysregulation. Train them to perceive mental contortions, like high contrast thinking, catastrophizing, or customizing, and help them reevaluate their considerations in a more adjusted and sensible manner. This can assist them with better dealing with their

feelings by changing their impression of circumstances.

5. Solid adapting abilities: Urge people with ADHD to foster sound adapting abilities to deal with their feelings. This can involve participating in active work, rehearsing care and contemplation, taking part in leisure activities or exercises they appreciate, conversing with a confidant companion or relative, or looking for proficient assistance from a specialist or guide. Solid adapting abilities can assist people with dealing with their feelings in a useful and sound way.

6. Breaks: Urge people with ADHD to enjoy reprieves when they notice their feelings rising. Getting some down time can offer them the chance to move back from the circumstance, take full breaths, and refocus prior to tending to the circumstance once more. This can assist with forestalling imprudent responses and take into account more smart and deliberate reactions.

7. Emotionally supportive network: Urge people with ADHD to construct an emotionally supportive network that incorporates confided in companions, relatives, or experts who can offer help and direction in dealing with their feelings. Having an emotionally supportive network can furnish people with ADHD with a place of refuge to communicate their feelings, get criticism, and gain point of view.

Seeking support when needed

Indeed, looking for help when required is critical for people with ADHD in dealing with their personal difficulties really. Here are a few contemplations for looking for help:

1. Specialist or guide: A certified psychological well-being proficient, like a specialist or advisor, can offer important help in assisting people with ADHD deal with their feelings. They can give methodologies, instruments, and procedures for profound guidelines, as well as a place of refuge to process and examine feelings. A specialist or

instructor can likewise assist people with creating solid survival strategies, distinguish triggers, and figure out through any hidden close to home problems that might be adding to their difficulties.

2. Support gatherings: Joining a care group for people with ADHD can be useful as it furnishes a chance to interface with other people who share comparable encounters. Support gatherings can offer approval, understanding, and viable ways to deal with feelings. It can likewise give a feeling of local area and diminish sensations of confinement.

3. Confided in loved ones: Having an emotionally supportive network of believed loved ones can be significant in dealing with feelings. These people can offer a listening ear, give compassion, and deal support during testing times. It's essential to discuss straightforwardly with confided in loved ones around one's feelings and look for their comprehension and backing.

4. School or work environment facilities:
    People with ADHD might profit from
    facilities at school or in the working
    environment to assist with dealing with
    their feelings really. This might
    incorporate changes to their current
    circumstance, for example, sound
    decrease measures, adaptable work
    hours, or extra breaks, as well as
    admittance to strong assets, like a guide
    or specialist.

5. Clinical experts: at times, people with
    ADHD might expect medicine to deal
    with their side effects, including inner
    difficulties. Talking with a certified
    clinical expert, like a therapist, can give
    significant bits of knowledge into drug
    choices and doses that can assist with
    close to home guidelines.

Chapter 10

Seeking Professional Help

Knowing when to seek professional help

Knowing when to look for proficient assistance is fundamental for people with ADHD. Here are a few signs that might show the requirement for proficient help:

1. Tenacious and huge impedance: On the off chance that ADHD side effects altogether influence a singular's everyday existence, like scholar or work execution, connections, or profound prosperity, in spite of their endeavors to oversee them, it could be an ideal opportunity to look for proficient assistance.

2. Trouble dealing with feelings: In the event that a person with ADHD encounters tireless trouble dealing with their feelings, for example, successive emotional episodes, serious close to

home explosions, or trouble controlling displeasure, bitterness, or tension, proficient help might be valuable.

3. Battling with connections: In the event that ADHD side effects are causing difficulties in connections, for example, successive struggles, trouble imparting, or issues with motivation control, looking for proficient assistance can give techniques and devices to really deal with these difficulties.

4. Debilitated personal satisfaction: In the event that ADHD side effects essentially influence a singular's general personal satisfaction, for example, disturbances in rest designs, trouble with using time effectively and association, disabled confidence, or decreased self-assurance, looking for proficient support might be useful.

5. Security concerns: In the event that a person with ADHD participates in unsafe ways of behaving, for example, substance misuse, imprudent or risky ways of behaving, or has contemplations of self-damage or self destruction, it's

basic to quickly look for proficient assistance.

6. Individual pain: In the event that a person with ADHD is encountering critical profound trouble, like wretchedness, tension, or constant sensations of overpower, it means quite a bit to look for proficient help to address these worries.

7. Absence of progress with self improvement systems: In the event that an individual has attempted self improvement procedures, for example, way of life changes, adapting methods, and other administration techniques, however isn't gaining critical headway in dealing with their ADHD side effects, looking for proficient assistance might be fundamental.

Understanding the different types of therapy for ADHD

There are a few sorts of treatment that can be helpful for people with ADHD. These may include:

1. Social treatment: Conduct treatment is a sort of treatment that spotlights on distinguishing and changing ways of behaving connected with ADHD side effects. It might include systems like putting forth objectives, laying out schedules, creating association and time usage abilities, and further developing motivation control. Conduct treatment can be especially powerful for youngsters and youths with ADHD, however it can likewise be useful for grown-ups.

2. Mental social treatment (CBT): Mental conduct treatment is a kind of treatment that spotlights the association between considerations, sentiments, and ways of behaving. It can assist people with ADHD distinguish and change pessimistic idea designs and foster survival techniques for overseeing ADHD side effects. CBT may likewise address co-happening conditions, for example, nervousness or sorrow, which are normal in people with ADHD.

3. Psychoeducation: Psychoeducation includes teaching people with ADHD

and their families about the condition, its side effects, and its effect on day to day existence. Psychoeducation can assist individuals with better figuring out their ADHD, master survival methods, and work on mindfulness.

4. Family treatment: Family treatment includes working with the whole family to further develop correspondence, understanding, and backing for the person with ADHD. It can assist families with creating techniques for overseeing ADHD-related difficulties at home, school, and in group environments, and can likewise address any relational peculiarities or clashes that might be affecting the person with ADHD.

5. Strong directing: Steady guiding can furnish people with ADHD a place of refuge to examine their considerations, sentiments, and concerns connected with their condition. It can assist people with handling feelings, work on confidence, and foster solid survival techniques.

6. Training: ADHD instructing includes working with an in mentor ADHD to lay out objectives, foster systems, and give responsibility to overseeing ADHD side effects. ADHD training can be especially useful for grown-ups with ADHD in further developing using time effectively, association, and efficiency abilities.

7. Medicine the executives: While not a customary type of treatment, prescription can be a significant part of ADHD treatment. Prescription, like energizer or non-energizer drugs, can assist with overseeing ADHD side effects and work on generally working. Drugs the board might be supervised by a specialist or other qualified medical care proficient.

Working with counselors or therapists for support

Working with advisors or specialists can be a significant piece of overseeing ADHD. Advisors and specialists can offer help, direction, and instruments for overseeing ADHD-related difficulties. Here are a few systems for successfully working with guides or specialists:

1. See as a certified proficient: Search for a guide or specialist who has insight and skill in working with people with ADHD. They ought to be authorized or affirmed in their field, and in a perfect world have experience working explicitly with ADHD clients.

2. Lay out clear objectives: Prior to beginning treatment, it's critical to lay out clear objectives for what you need to accomplish. Talk about your particular worries connected with ADHD, for example, overseeing side effects, further developing using time productively, association, adapting to inner difficulties, or further developing connections. Team up with your guide or advisor to lay out sensible and feasible objectives for treatment.

3. Convey transparently and truly: Be transparent with your instructor or advisor about your ADHD side effects, difficulties, and concerns. Share your contemplations, sentiments, and encounters connected with ADHD, as well as some other emotional wellness or close to home worries you might have. This will assist your instructor or advisor with better figuring out your necessities and designing the treatment to your particular circumstance.

4. Completely finish suggestions: Your advisor or specialist might furnish you with proposals or techniques for overseeing ADHD side effects or further developing adapting abilities. Finishing these suggestions and carrying them out in your everyday routine is significant. Be focused on effectively captivating in treatment and rehearsing the abilities acquired during meetings.

5. Team up on systems and procedures: Work cooperatively with your advisor or specialist to foster methodologies and strategies that work for you. This might incorporate creating adapting abilities

for overseeing impulsivity, further developing using time productively and association, overseeing pressure, and controlling feelings. Be available to attempt new methodologies and give input to your guide or advisor on what works and what doesn't.

6. Practice taking care of oneself: Overseeing ADHD can be testing, and focusing on taking care of oneself is significant. This might incorporate getting sufficient rest, eating a reasonable eating routine, participating in customary actual activity, and rehearsing unwinding strategies. Your instructor or specialist can assist you with fostering a taking care of oneself arrangement that upholds your general prosperity.

7. Be predictable and committed: Overseeing ADHD takes time and exertion, and progress may not be quick. Be predictable and focused on going to treatment meetings routinely, executing suggested procedures, and rehearsing new abilities reliably in your everyday existence. Recall that change requires

some investment, and show restraint toward yourself as you pursue your objectives.

8. Look for extra help when required: In the event that you feel that you want extra help past directing or treatment, like prescription administration, training, or different administrations, examine this with your advocate or specialist. They can assist you with investigating fitting choices and make references on a case by case basis.

Incorporating professional help as part of self-care routine

Consolidating proficient assistance as a component of your taking care of oneself routine can be a proactive step towards dealing with your ADHD really. Here are a few procedures for integrating proficient assistance into your taking care of oneself daily practice:

1. Perceive the significance of expert assistance: Figure out that looking for proficient assistance, like guiding,

treatment, training, or drug the board, is definitely not an indication of shortcoming, but instead a proactive step towards overseeing ADHD. Perceive that overseeing ADHD can be testing, and looking for proficient assistance can furnish you with the help, instruments, and methodologies you really want to adapt to the difficulties successfully.

2. Focus on it: Very much like you focus on different parts of taking care of oneself, like rest, nourishment, and exercise, focus on proficient assistance as a feature of your taking care of oneself daily schedule. Plan customary meetings with your guide, specialist, or different experts, and focus on going to these arrangements in your timetable.

3. View as the right proficient: Finding the right proficient who grasps ADHD and has insight in working with people with ADHD is essential. Do all necessary investigation, request suggestions from confided in sources, and interview possible experts to guarantee they are ideal for your necessities.

4. Team up with experts: Whenever you have seen as an expert, effectively participate during the time spent working with them. Team up with them on defining objectives, creating procedures, and carrying out methods to really deal with your ADHD side effects. Be available to criticism, seek clarification on pressing issues, and effectively partake in the treatment or training process.

5. Execute suggested methodologies: Experts might give you proposals, procedures, or strategies for overseeing ADHD side effects or further developing adapting abilities. Be focused on carrying out these proposals in your everyday daily practice. Practice and coordinate the procedures into your day to day existence every time to see positive outcomes.

6. Convey straightforwardly and truly: Be transparent with your experts about your side effects, difficulties, and concerns. Share your contemplations, sentiments, and encounters connected

with ADHD, as well as some other psychological wellness or close to home worries you might have. This will assist them with better grasping your requirements and designing their way to deal with your particular circumstance.

7. Completely finish proposals: It's essential to totally finish the suggestions given by your experts. This might incorporate going to customary arrangements, accepting recommended drugs as coordinated, and executing procedures or methods mastered during treatment or training meetings. Consistency and responsibility are vital to seeing positive outcomes.

8. Practice self-reflection and mindfulness: As a component of your taking care of oneself daily schedule, practice self-reflection and mindfulness. Focus on your viewpoints, sentiments, ways of behaving, and sets off connected with ADHD. Routinely evaluate your advancement, recognize regions that might require improvement, and convey them to your experts to make vital

changes in accordance with your treatment plan.

9. Advocate for yourself: Be a functioning supporter for yourself in your cooperations with experts. Be self-assured in communicating your necessities, concerns, and inclinations. Request explanation or extra data when required, and effectively take part in choices connected with your treatment plan.

10. Look for extra help when required: Assuming you feel that you want extra help past your ongoing expert assistance, make sure to do it. This might incorporate contacting different experts, support gatherings, or confiding in people in your day to day existence. It's OK to look for extra help depending on the situation to guarantee you are successfully dealing with your ADHD and dealing with your emotional well-being.

Conclusion

In conclusion, "Self Care for Teens with ADHD" is a comprehensive guide that emphasizes the importance of self-care for the overall well-being of teenagers with ADHD. Throughout this book, we have explored various strategies and techniques for teens to effectively manage their ADHD symptoms, improve their mental health, and enhance their quality of life.

From understanding the unique challenges of ADHD in teens to learning practical self-care strategies, this book has covered a wide range of topics, including healthy lifestyle habits, stress management techniques, emotional regulation skills, and strategies for enhancing focus and attention. We have also discussed the importance of building a supportive network, seeking professional help when needed, and developing a positive mindset towards ADHD.

It is our hope that this book has provided valuable insights, practical tips, and encouragement for teens with ADHD to take charge of their well-being and thrive despite the challenges they may face. We have emphasized that self-care is not selfish, but rather a necessary investment in one's physical, mental, and emotional health. By prioritizing self-care and implementing the strategies discussed in this book, teens with ADHD can develop resilience, improve their mental health, and lead a fulfilling life.

Remember, managing ADHD is a journey, and self-care is a continuous process. It requires effort, commitment, and support from both the individual and their support system. We encourage teens with ADHD to be patient with themselves, celebrate their progress, and seek help when needed. With the right strategies and mindset, teens with ADHD can take charge of their well-being and lead a meaningful, fulfilling life.

We hope that "Self Care for Teens with ADHD" has been a valuable resource in empowering teens with ADHD to prioritize self-care and take control of their mental health and overall well-being. May this book serve as a guide to support and inspire teens with ADHD on their journey to managing their condition and living a fulfilling life. Remember, you are not alone, and you have the power to thrive with ADHD by practicing self-care and taking charge of your well-being.